# HOW
# EASE
# ANXIETY

### Embrace Calm and Say Goodbye
### to Worries for Good

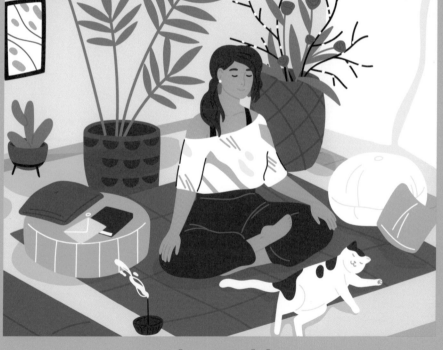

## Sophie Golding

HOW TO EASE YOUR ANXIETY

Text by Kitiara Pascoe

An Hachette UK Company
www.hachette.co.uk

Vie Books, an imprint of Summersdale Publishers
Part of Octopus Publishing Group Limited
Carmelite House
50 Victoria Embankment
LONDON
EC4Y 0DZ
UK

www.summersdale.com

Printed and bound in China

ISBN: 978-1-83799-379-6

Substantial discounts on bulk quantities of Summersdale books are available to corporations, professional associations and other organizations. For details contact general enquiries: telephone: +44 (0) 1243 771107 or email: enquiries@summersdale.com.

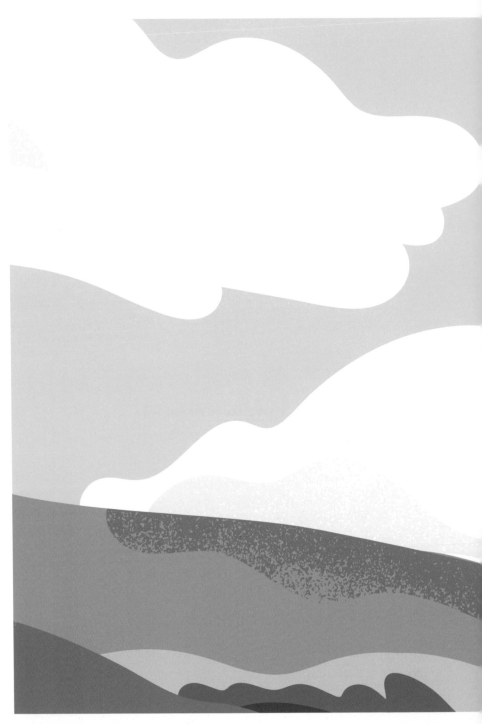

# INTRODUCTION

Almost everybody experiences anxiety at some point. It's a perfectly natural feeling that might appear before you step on stage for a big performance or ask your significant other to marry you, for instance. For some of us, though, it arises in everyday situations too, such as getting into the car or calling a restaurant to make a reservation. If we find ourselves avoiding something because of our anxiety, we will likely miss out on parts of life that can be truly enriching. Learning to recognize, observe and work with anxiety is vital in order to start living life on our own terms.

This book will help you recognize anxious thoughts and feelings and learn how to approach them, so that even when you experience challenges, you'll have the tools to manage them and live the life you want. By picking up this book, you've already started your journey to anxiety-free living. As you work your way towards the final pages, you will hopefully feel happier and more confident and have a greater sense of freedom in your life. Are you ready? Let's dive in!

# CHAPTER ONE

# WHAT DOES ANXIETY LOOK LIKE?

For some people, anxiety is unmistakable, while for others, it might come as an "Ah ha!" moment when they hear a description of its characteristics. Perhaps you recognize it fluttering in your stomach before a meeting, or when you feel nauseous for seemingly no reason. Or maybe you've found yourself turning down the chance to try a new experience that sounds quite fun, because of worry or uncertainty. Perhaps you've stepped back from opportunities when you wish you could have stepped forwards. Anxiety can show up in many forms, and learning to recognize it is the first step to managing and moving past it.

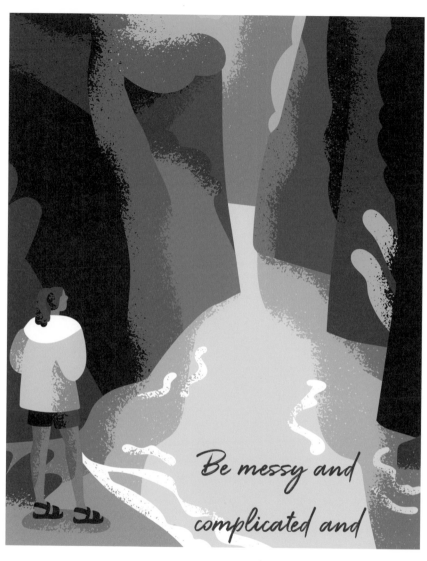

Be messy and
complicated and
afraid and show
up anyway.

Glennon Doyle

# HOW TO SPOT
# SIGNS OF ANXIETY

Anxiety isn't a one-size-fits-all experience, and its intensity can vary from hour to hour, day to day or even year to year. It can manifest in the form of physical symptoms as well as mental ones, and these symptoms may change or even develop a pattern. Often, anxiety can be low-level, but it can also be the cause of more disruptive symptoms. Here's a small selection:

- Faster or more noticeable heartbeat
- Sweating that's not due to heat
- Pins and needles
- Discomfort or pain in the chest
- Racing, intrusive thoughts
- Ruminating on past incidents or conversations
- Avoiding situations that may cause anxiety

If you experience one of the above symptoms, consider what situation you're in or what you're thinking about at the time. Getting into the habit of spotting anxiety means you can take action to manage it more quickly, before it becomes too disruptive – for example, by focusing on the present (page 52) or by jotting down a few things you're grateful for (page 74).

# EVERYONE IS DIFFERENT, EVERYONE IS WORTHY

A common thought when considering your experience with anxiety (or its cousin, depression) is wondering whether yours is "bad enough". But anxiety is triggered in different people for different reasons, and the symptoms can vary from one person to another. If you feel you experience anxiety on a lower level to someone else, that's no reason to dismiss or diminish it. However your anxiety is manifesting, it's very real to you and needs attention. Try to be kind and considerate of your own experiences.

You don't have to control your thoughts; you just have to stop letting them control you.

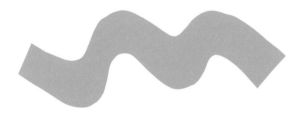

**Dan Millman**

# A FREER FUTURE

Knowing why you want to manage your anxiety will help keep you on track. Find a quiet place and grab a pen and paper. Then write down what reducing your anxiety will mean for you, using "I can" and "I will" statements. For example:

- "I will be able to go to my friends' parties and meet new people."
- "I can drive my family where they need to go and be more generous with my time."
- "I will share my expertise in meetings."

Take a moment to picture yourself in each scenario, free from anxiety. How will it feel?

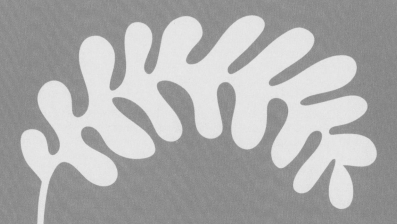

Strength
resonates
within me

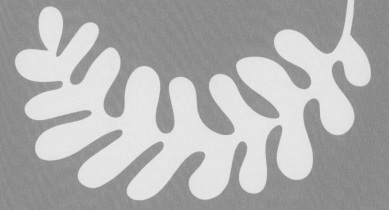

# A "MISSED OPPORTUNITY" INVENTORY

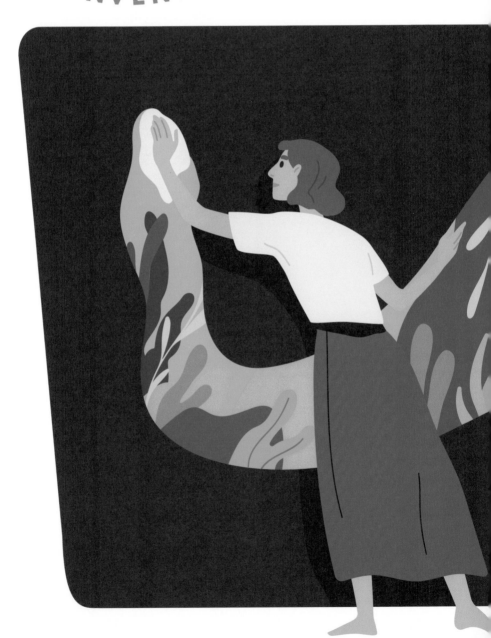

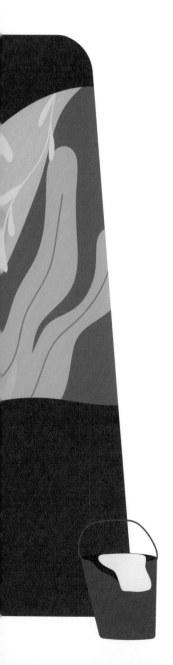

A great first step in taking stock of how anxiety affects you is to reflect on how it may have led to missed opportunities. This is a hopeful exercise that helps you see why you might have made decisions in the past that disappoint you, and how you can prevent anxiety from stopping you in the future.

**When was anxiety steering you?** Get comfy with a pen and paper, and let your mind wander over the past. Can you think of any opportunities you wish you'd had the "confidence" to seize? Sometimes, when we think we lack confidence, it's actually anxiety that has taken the wheel. Here are some nudges:

• You wanted to ask for a raise, but, at the end of your appraisal, you stopped yourself from speaking up.

• Your friend invited you to the gym, but you declined as you worried people might stare.

• You struggled to enjoy an activity because you kept thinking about a negative comment someone made the day before.

Write down any missed opportunities that come to mind, big or small. It's time to forgive yourself for them and to recognize that anxiety likely played the leading role.

The key to realizing
a dream is to focus
not on success but
on significance –

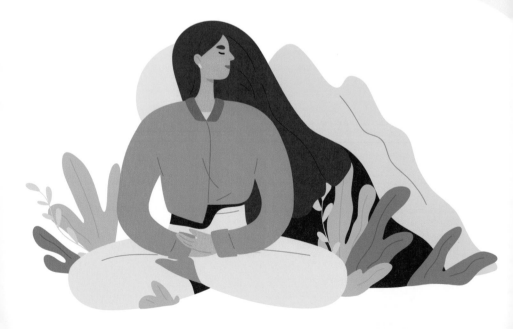

and then even the small
steps and little victories
along your path will
take on greater meaning.

**Oprah Winfrey**

# FLIPPING ENVY ON ITS HEAD

The way we react to other people can be a golden ticket to understanding our true feelings. Do you ever feel uncomfortable when hearing about someone else's achievements? Do you find yourself saying or thinking something negative about another's success? Reflect on moments when you've experienced these difficult feelings and consider what you might really have been responding to. It's often not about the person or the achievement at all - rather, these feelings are highlighting a perceived lack or insecurity that we hold within. Discovering these gives us awareness, and with awareness comes the power to change.

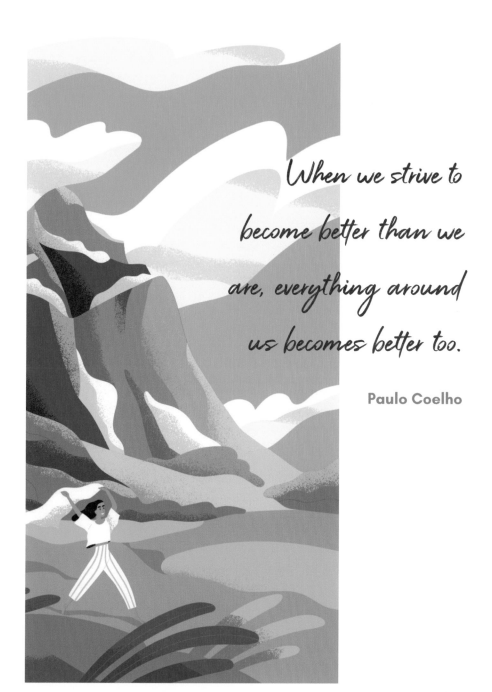

When we strive to become better than we are, everything around us becomes better too.

Paulo Coelho

# CONTENTS

# LIFE IS NOT
# PAINT-BY-NUMBERS

Perhaps your friends have made big life choices or reached "milestones" you haven't. If this is the case, it's all too easy to feel as though you're behind. Anxiety can crop up fast when you start counting all the things you haven't yet done. But this is your life, nobody else's, and you get to choose which direction you go and when. Create one or two go-to mantras for when you feel like you're not "keeping up". For example:

- I am exactly where I should be.
- Every day, I am progressing on my unique journey.

I'm excited to see where
my life leads me...
and where I lead my life

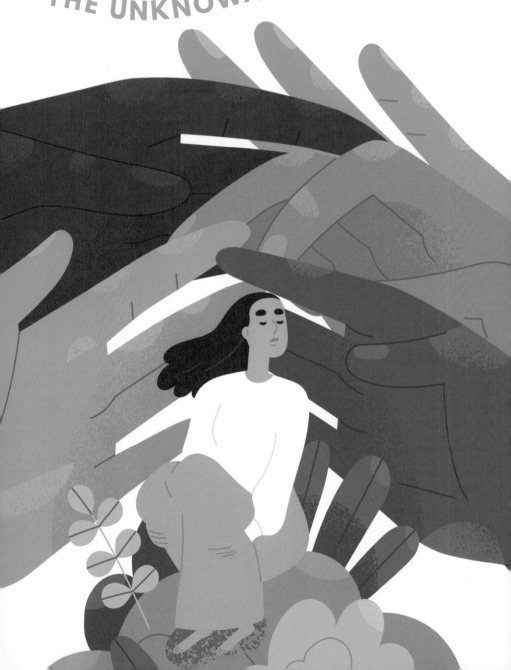

TRYING TO KNOW
THE UNKNOWABLE

The easiest things to do are usually the things you do most often: the familiar. It's the unknown that most often triggers anxiety, be it a new job, a new route to drive, a sea of unfamiliar faces at a party or not knowing where a conversation might head.

Some people become experts at planning and organization not because these are useful skills to have, but because of anxiety. Being highly organized is one thing, but if you are ultra-organized because the idea of not knowing what will happen brings feelings of dread and anxiety, it's important to pay attention.

Take a moment to think of classic anxiety triggers for you (going to an event where you don't know anyone, for example), and imagine that you know exactly what will happen, or what the conversation will be, or what you need to do and say in that situation. Does that scenario now seem more manageable? If so, it might not be the precise situation that triggers your anxiety, but the unknown variables within it.

# A WEEKLY SHADOW

Anxious thoughts can arrive for many reasons, but most people usually have particular recurrent ones. One of the first steps when addressing anxiety is to examine your most frequent triggers – this is where you can make the biggest change. Consider your average day or week, then write down any recurring situations that cause anxiety. For example:

- A weekly presentation
  - The route you drive every Thursday
    - Your gym sessions

When it comes to learning techniques or getting specific help, understanding your recurring triggers is a good place to start.

You can't plough a field
by turning it over in your
mind. To begin, begin.

**Gordon B. Hinckley**

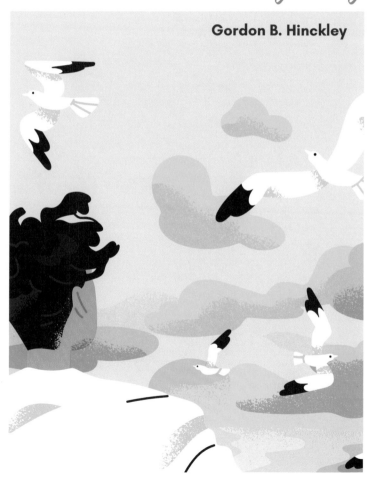

# THINK ABOUT WHAT YOU DRINK

Coffee is a go-to drink for many, but its caffeine content is a common contributor to anxiety. The amount of caffeine in coffee can vary widely, and the way your body responds to it can change, too, due to the rate your body metabolizes caffeine.

To see whether caffeine is playing a role in anxiety, you could start a "jitter journal". Note down when you drink caffeinated coffee each day and how you feel during the hours afterwards. Reduce your intake and see if you start recording lower anxiety levels in your journal. Why not rethink that double-shot espresso hidden in your mug and try a caffeine-free herbal tea instead?

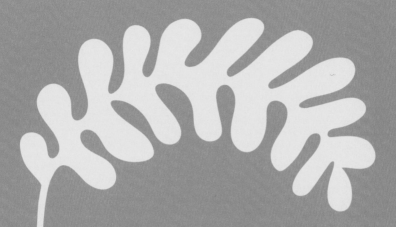

My thoughts
shape my world

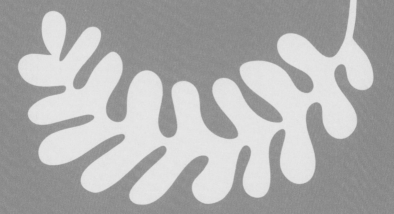

# WHO'S THE IMPOSTER?

If you've ever felt as though you're not good enough to do something - even though you meet the standards on paper - you're in good company. Huge numbers of people experience "imposter syndrome" - a feeling of not deserving their position and worrying that someone will find them out. This can prevent you from applying for jobs or promotions, seeing your achievements in a true light, or fully stepping into your personal power. Consider these questions:

- Have you ever minimized your achievements when praised?
- Do you deny being knowledgeable about something, even when you are?
- Have you ever opted out of something because you thought you weren't good enough?

Recognizing imposter syndrome is an important step in dealing with this very common strand of anxiety. When you can see it's played a part in some of your decisions, actions or conversations, then you can start learning techniques to manage it, such as saying "no" (page 36) and showing yourself greater respect (page 136).

I can say "yes" to things I want

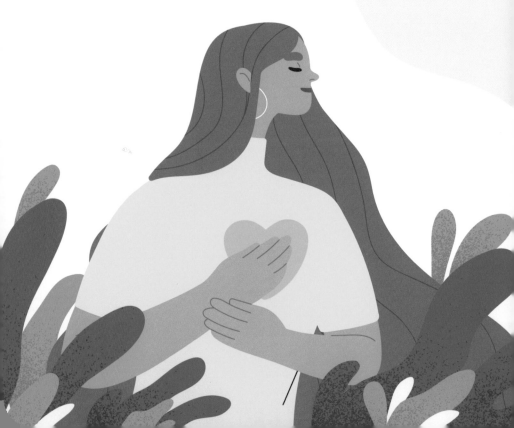

*and "no" to things*

*that do not serve me*

# PERFORM A "BRAIN DUMP"

Left to their own devices, worries will bounce around your head endlessly. Getting them out of your brain and onto paper nails them down where you can deal with them! Try keeping a notepad to hand (or use a notes app on your phone), so that when you notice anxiety cropping up you can briefly write down what's on your mind. Seeing it in black and white can help reduce its weight and power. For example, "I'm having friends over for dinner, but I'm worried there won't be enough food." Read the worries back to yourself and perhaps they'll seem smaller, or you might even spot an easy solution.

*I will be calm.*

*I will be mistress*

*of myself.*

**Jane Austen**

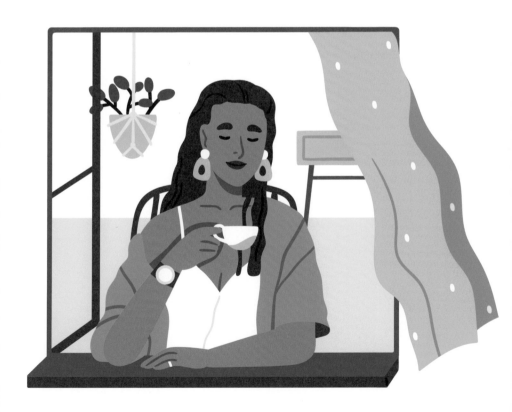

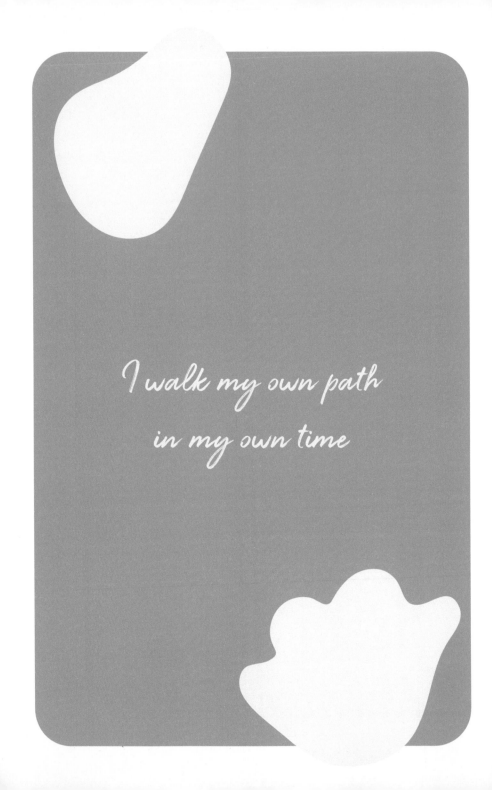

I walk my own path
in my own time

# Don't let someone else's opinion of you become your reality.

**Les Brown**

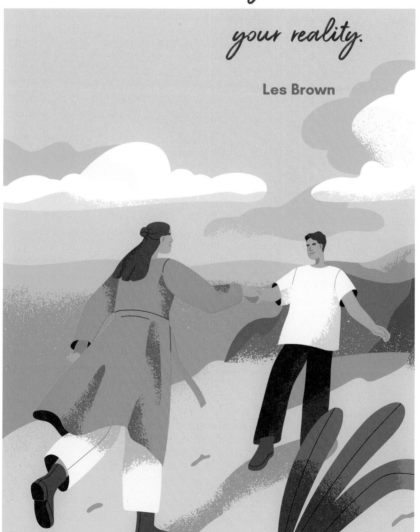

# THE POWER OF "NO"

It's natural to want to help others and make a good impression, but when you find yourself repeatedly saying "yes" to things you don't want – or don't have time – to do, anxiety can be both the cause and the result.

Saying "yes" because you're worried there'll be negative repercussions by being honest can be an anxiety-driven habit. But becoming overloaded is a surefire path to extra stress and worry. Try saying "no" to small things first and see how your confidence grows when you become more intentional about what you agree to.

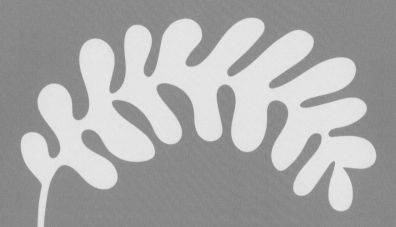

Hold your
boundaries firm

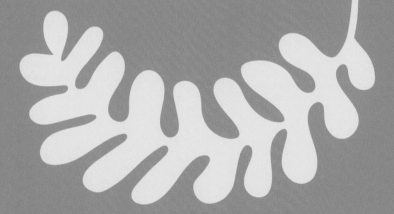

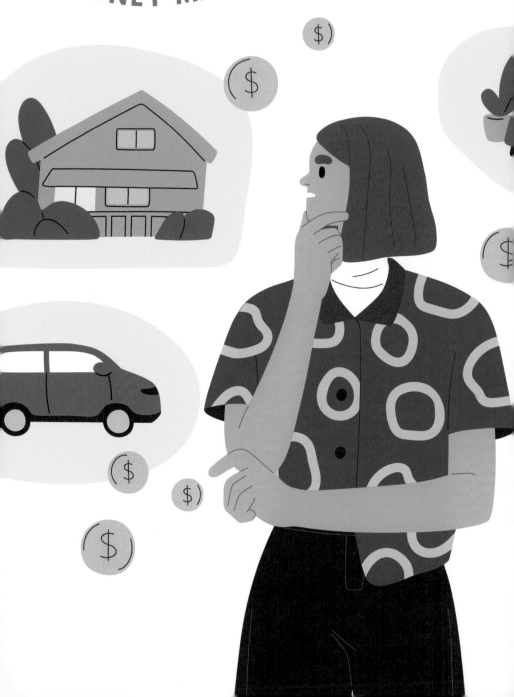

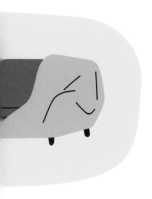

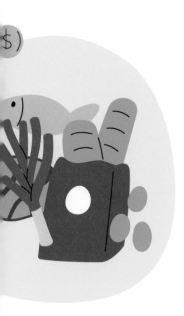

Few things in life are as anxiety-inducing as money, so it's important to acknowledge these concerns if they factor into your life. It's useful to seek financial advice from banks, charities or local authorities, but when do these feelings tip from being a little worrying to full-on financial anxiety? Here are some common markers:

- Being unable to bring yourself to look at your bank balance

- Hiding your financial situation from your partner or family

- Beating yourself up over purchases or past spending decisions

- Constantly thinking about money and your finances

As most people don't discuss their finances with friends or even family, it's easy to stay isolated and lose perspective on this topic. You don't need to be struggling for money to feel financial anxiety, either: financially comfortable people can also find themselves losing sleep over money worries. The first thing to do is recognize you have some anxiety around money and decide to take control of it. Throughout this book, you'll find tips and tools that will help you regain power in your life, such as visualization exercises (page 122).

*Courage starts with showing up and letting ourselves be seen.*

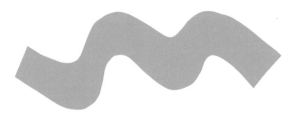

**Brené Brown**

# YOUR PRESENCE IS VALUED

A racing heart rate and intrusive thoughts are big hitters when it comes to anxiety, but worries can show up in more subtle ways, too. Have you ever found yourself not replying to a friend who wants to meet up, or not RSVPing to an event? Perhaps you think you won't be missed at the party, or that your friend has better things to do than see you. Always remember, you are loved and valued by your friends, and an invitation means that someone would love to have your company. Take a moment to focus on that mutual love, and reflect it back in your response, even if you can't go.

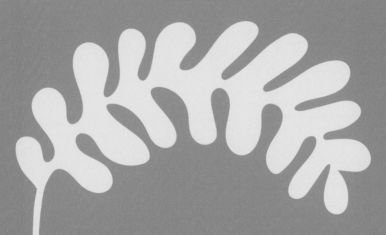

I embrace
failure and
stride forwards
with my new
knowledge

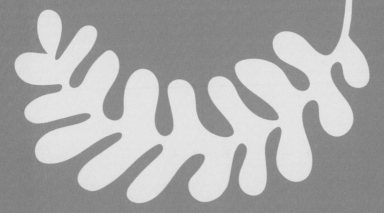

# FAILURE IS THE PATH TO PROGRESS

Anxiety often rears its head any time there's a possibility you might fail. Failure could mean getting rejected on a date, someone not laughing at your joke, having no customers for your business... any multitude of things. Acknowledging that you experience a fear of failure is an important step in managing anxiety, as is accepting there's nothing wrong with this fear. The next step is to consciously remind yourself that failure is the path to progress and success. Without failure, we would never learn how to adapt or improve – plus, it's an important part of developing resilience. Failure is a powerful tool that helps propel us along the right path.

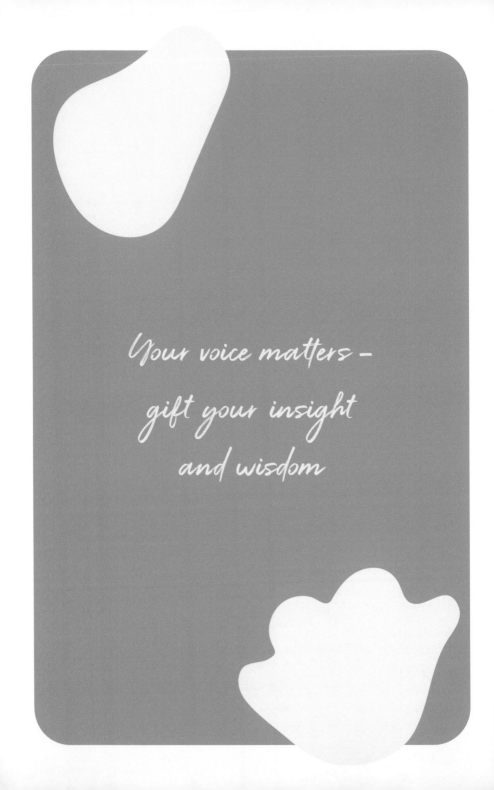

Your voice matters –
gift your insight
and wisdom

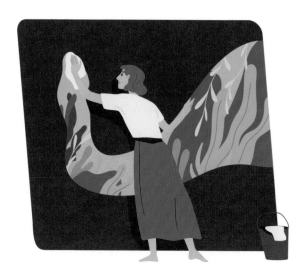

# CHAPTER TWO

# BE KIND TO YOUR MIND

How you treat yourself is exceptionally important when it comes to dealing with the stressors life throws at you, so it's vital you build solid mental foundations. Anxious thoughts usually follow a pattern, and a mind used to berating itself will have few defences against them. Being kind to your mind, and supporting it with healthy habits and practices, is one of the best things you can do to manage anxiety and live a happy, stable life. It helps build resilience and wisdom, so you know that, whatever happens – both the good and the bad – you will be okay.

# THE FRIEND TEST

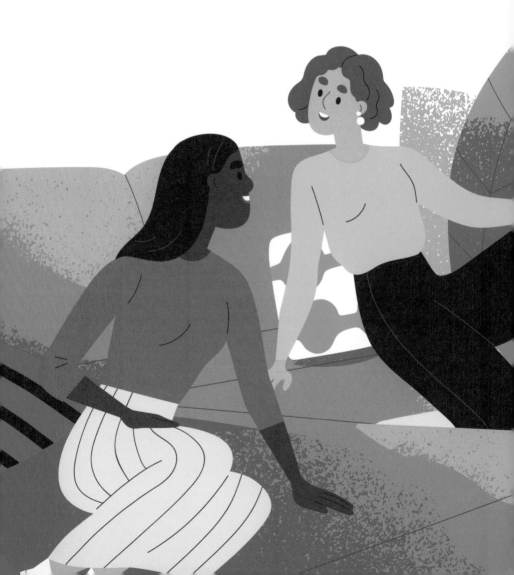

Imagine you were going to have a person by your side every second of your life. You'd probably want them to be friendly and supportive, right? The truth is, you do have a person with you all the time - you. The friend test is a great way to begin spotting where you could be kinder to yourself.

Think about how you speak to yourself on a daily basis. What do you think when you look in the mirror or walk away from a chat with a senior colleague? What do you say to yourself when you try on clothes that don't suit you? Would you say any of those things to a friend? If your self-talk is negative, chances are, you wouldn't dream of it.

Jot down a few key phrases you often level against yourself. Now, write the version you would say to your best friend. Next time you catch yourself saying unfriendly things to yourself, opt for the kinder version instead. It's a small change that can have a huge impact.

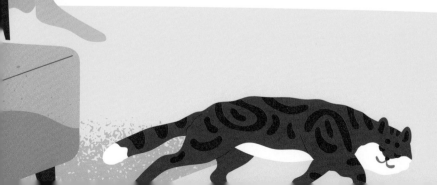

# SEE SOCIAL MEDIA
# FOR WHAT IT IS

Images on social media are seldom any more "real" than images in magazines. They're curated in a way that gives a certain impression and, when that's all you see, it's easy to believe that person is always laughing on a beach or rocking incredible hair. Consider how each social media app makes you feel and why you end up scrolling through it. Simply drawing your awareness to this is the first step. Then, try muting or unfollowing accounts that make you feel less than, and consider limiting your usage by opting for social-media-free days.

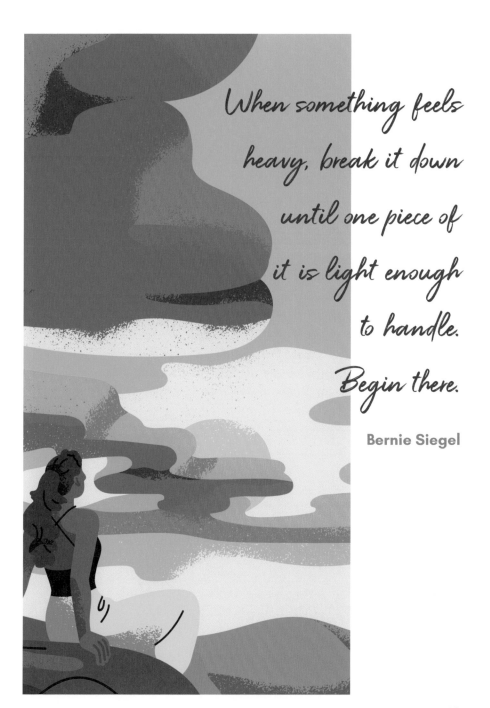

When something feels
heavy, break it down
until one piece of
it is light enough
to handle.
Begin there.

**Bernie Siegel**

# RECITE MORNING MANTRAS

Start each day the way you mean to go on – with kindness and positivity. Write a short list of supportive, positive mantras and stick it somewhere you'll definitely see, such as in your bathroom or on your wardrobe door. Mantras could include "I am filled with light and energy", or "Great things await me today". Pick one mantra every day and say it out loud in front of a mirror. It might sound like too small a habit to make a difference, but starting your day like this can put you in a better frame of mind, no matter what happens.

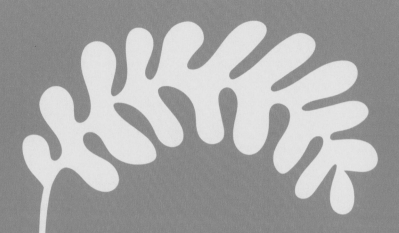

I see and
appreciate
the wonder
in every day

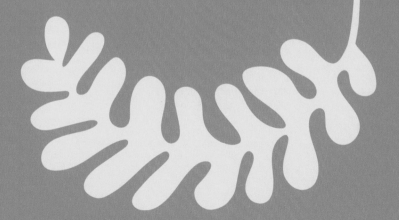

# REMAIN PEACEFULLY PRESENT

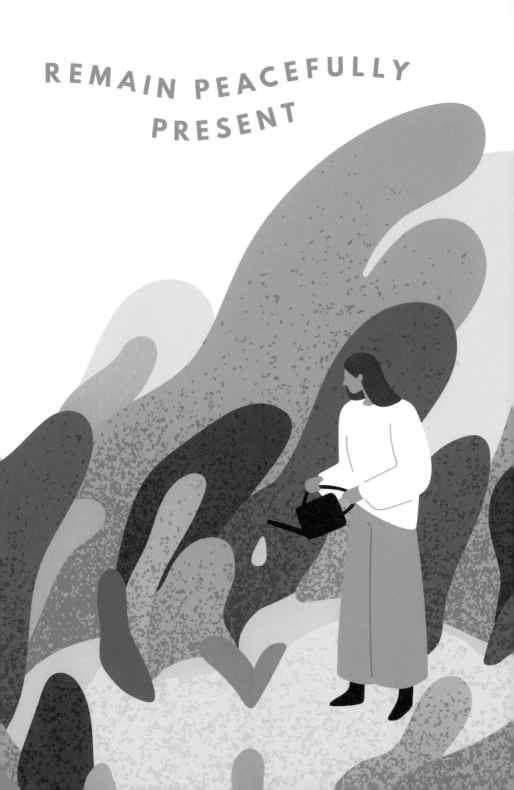

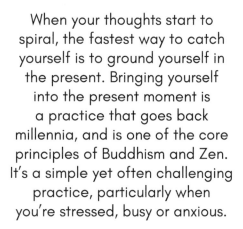

When your thoughts start to spiral, the fastest way to catch yourself is to ground yourself in the present. Bringing yourself into the present moment is a practice that goes back millennia, and is one of the core principles of Buddhism and Zen. It's a simple yet often challenging practice, particularly when you're stressed, busy or anxious.

Getting present can be done anywhere, at any time. Here are some ways to focus your mind in the present and quiet the chaos:

• Focus on touch. Think about how your feet rest on the ground, the texture of an item of clothing you're wearing, or simply touch your hands together, paying great attention to how this feels.

• Focus on breath. Breathe in for a count of four, pause, then exhale for a count of four. Practising calm, steady breathing is a fast way to the present.

• Focus on scent, sight or sound. Pick one sense and concentrate on it. What can you smell, see or hear right now? This prevents your mind from thinking about anything but what you're trying to sense.

I promise you nothing
is as chaotic as it
seems. Nothing is worth
diminishing your health.

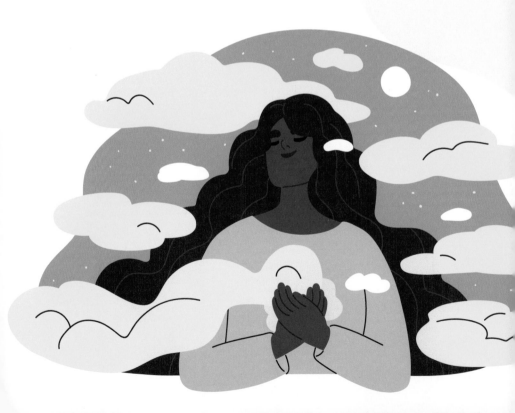

*Nothing is worth poisoning yourself into stress, anxiety, and fear.*

**Steve Maraboli**

# YOUR BEST IS GOOD ENOUGH

The phrase "You can only do your best" is as true now as it was when you were six years old. Except you can take it further and remind yourself: "You can only do the best you can with the energy and information you have at the time". The concept of "your best" can change daily – even hourly – and depends on everything from your workload and lunch choice to illness and weather conditions. Remind yourself often that you're doing the best you can and this is enough.

*Don't be afraid.*

*Be focused.*

*Be determined.*

*Be hopeful.*

*Be empowered.*

**Michelle Obama**

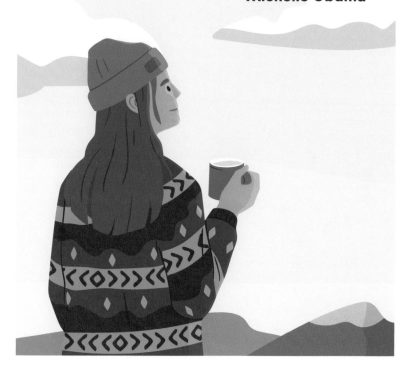

# TAKE FIVE
# FULL BREATHS

It's amazing how just five full breaths can transform how you feel. You could do this exercise every morning, or during the day whenever you need a restorative pause to recentre yourself:

- Sit comfortably and close your eyes, or keep your gaze soft.
- Inhale slowly, filling your lungs to the top.
- Exhale slowly.
- Repeat four more times.

Pause and appreciate the quiet before moving on to the rest of your day.

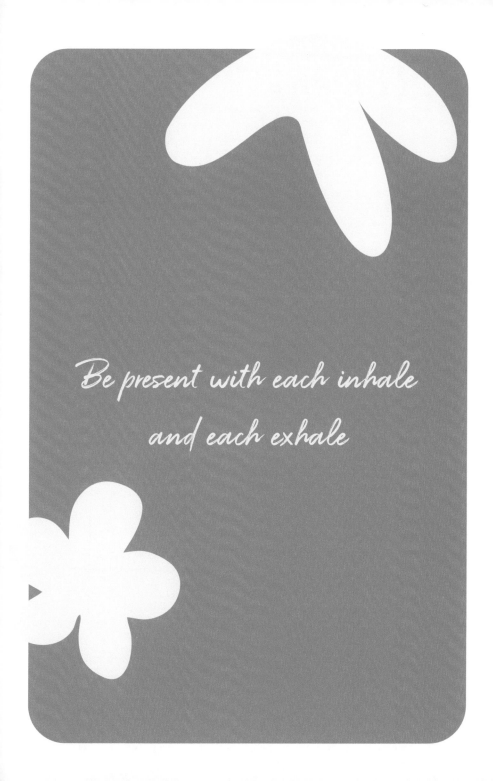

Be present with each inhale
and each exhale

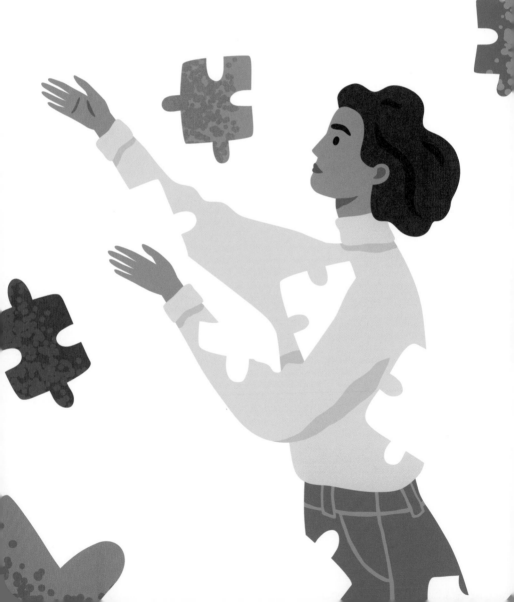

THE PAST CAN
BE STICKY

The past can be a source of learning, humour and nostalgia. But if certain events keep running through your head, making you feel like you can't change or keeping you trapped in the same patterns, it's overstepped the mark.

### Accept and forgive

Accepting that what's happened has happened is vital for moving on. To do this, we often have to forgive ourselves for our part in it, whether it's forgiveness for something we did, or for something we didn't do.

### Learn from past events

A healthy way to work with the past is to learn from it, rather than be held back by it. Lessons might be something actionable, like "I will be better prepared in that situation next time", or something supportive, like "I survived it, I am strong".

### Shape your environment

People, places and objects can keep us stuck in the past. Do you own something that reminds you of past negativity? Consider getting rid of it. Does a location or person keep drawing you backwards? Try visiting new places, experiencing new things and either branching out in your social life or letting the person know that you want to move forwards.

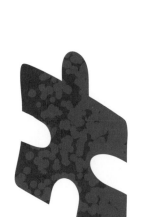
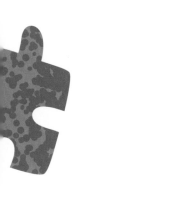
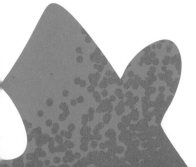

# SEEK OUT JOY EVERY DAY

When you look for joy in each day, you will find it, which can help to ease anxiety. It can take some practice to begin noticing things and letting yourself feel little eruptions of happiness. The things that bring people pockets of joy can be unique, but here are some suggestions of what to pay attention to:

- Birds singing, hopping about or fluffing up their feathers
- Hearing a great song
- Sharing a joke with a stranger in a shop
- Opening a new book
- Getting into a freshly made bed

When you give joy to other people, you get more joy in return. You should give a good thought to happiness that you can give out.

**Eleanor Roosevelt**

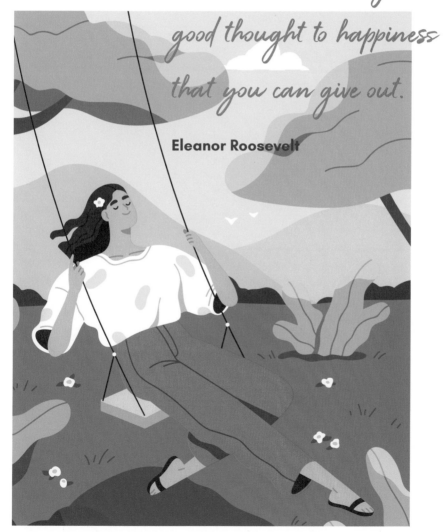

# ENGAGE IN POSITIVE ACTIVITIES

Anxiety can turn your brain into a tangled ball of wool, distracting you from your job and family and taking up far more time than you have to give. A great way to lighten the load temporarily is to give your mind something else – something positive – to focus on:

- Read a gripping novel.
- Watch a stand-up comedy special (or choose a short video if you're short on time).
- If you play an instrument, go through a few favourite pieces.
- Write a haiku (it doesn't have to be good!).

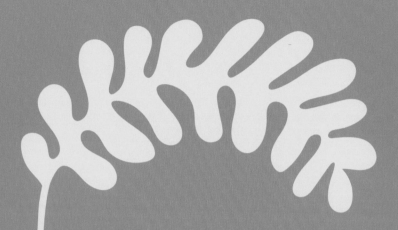

Laugh often
- it will help to
lighten the load

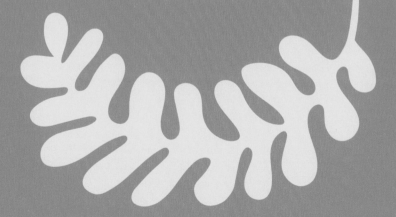

# KNOW YOUR
# BOUNDARIES

When you're feeling anxious, particularly in relation to others, you might find yourself saying "yes" to things you wish you hadn't. Perhaps you worry what people will think if you turn down a work project or social event. Maybe you have a friend who always asks for favours and you find yourself saying "yes" resentfully. We all have natural boundaries, but a lifetime of people pleasing can make our limits difficult to see and defend.

### Reframe the idea of boundaries
When you turn something down or protect your free time, you're not letting anybody down. You're shielding your energy so you can better apply it to your priorities, which might be another person, project or downtime.

### Get comfortable with "no"
When you always say "yes" to people, it starts to lose its power and you can find your time taken for granted. Saying "no" more often gives far more meaning to your "yes" when you do say it.

### Taking care of yourself
When you're exhausted, run down or resentful, you can't bring your full energy to anything. Prioritizing self-kindness helps protect your boundaries and keeps your energy topped up.

The tough times, the
days when you're just
a ball on the floor –

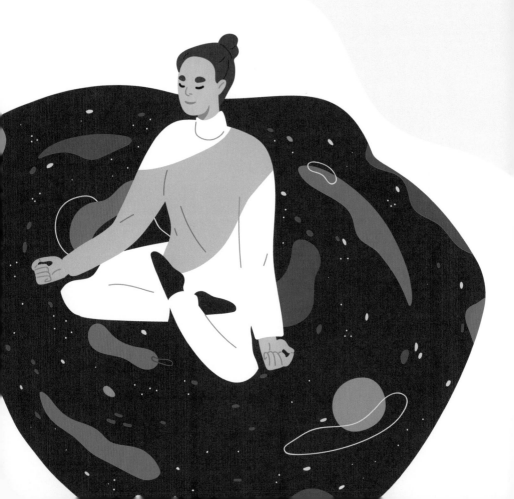

they'll pass. You're playing the long game, and life is totally worth it.

Sarah Silverman

# TAKE A
# REALITY
# CHECK

Remember when your parents told you not to believe everything you read? That's never been more true than today. It's astounding how realistic images enhanced and generated with artificial intelligence can be – from having vastly amplified colours to perfect skin and hair.

A simple way to alleviate status- or appearance-driven anxiety is to remind yourself often that what you see in adverts, magazines, online and even in films is not real. The images don't reflect what that person looks like in real life, the sky wasn't that blue and the leaves weren't that golden. You're not doing anything wrong if your life doesn't match those images: your life is real.

*I think it's just as important what you say no to as what you say yes to.*

**Sandra Oh**

# YOU ARE YOUR
# GREATEST ASSET

Anxiety has a habit of making us feel like we're not good enough – that we'll say the wrong thing, wear the wrong thing or generally be "not right". You don't have to apologize for being you, though: it's your individuality that makes you so wonderful. Studies have shown that diverse teams make stronger companies, as the individuals bring a greater range of background knowledge and experience. So be yourself, proudly: anything else is a disservice to you and the people around you.

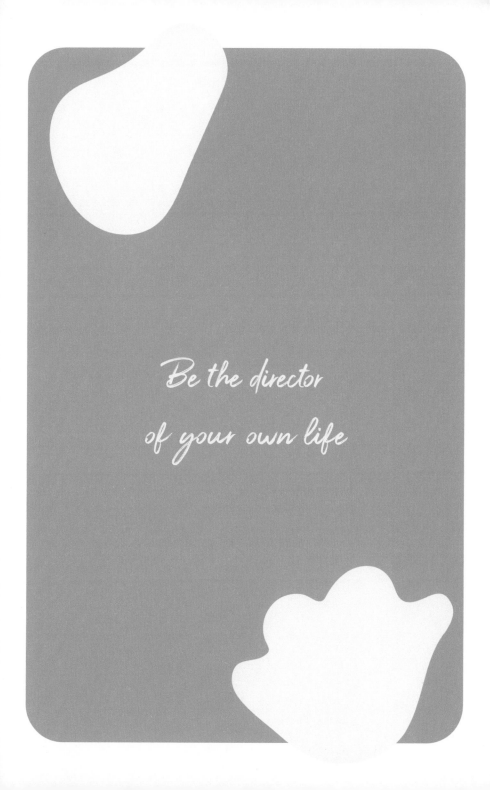

Be the director
of your own life

# GRATITUDE WILL
# LIFT YOU HIGHER

The anxious mind likes to focus on the negatives, so it can feel like every day is filled with challenges, fear or bad luck. While it's natural for negative occurrences to feature more prominently in the memory, you can train your mind to spot positivity too. The more you do it, the more easily and naturally it will come. Keeping a gratitude journal is an excellent way to achieve this. Before long, you'll see that your days have plenty of good things in them.

### Starting a gratitude practice
Choose a notebook or place on your phone where you'll jot down the things you're grateful for. Consistency is key, so having a set place to write is best.

### Just a few things
Every day, write down a few things you appreciate. Perhaps they happened during the day, or maybe they're broader than that - for example, the sun coming out at lunchtime or having kind and friendly neighbours.

### Notice a lightness
When you've written your list, consider how you feel. A little lighter, perhaps? Gratitude does wonders for uplifting the mood.

Do not anticipate
trouble or worry about
what may never happen.
Keep in the sunlight.

**Benjamin Franklin**

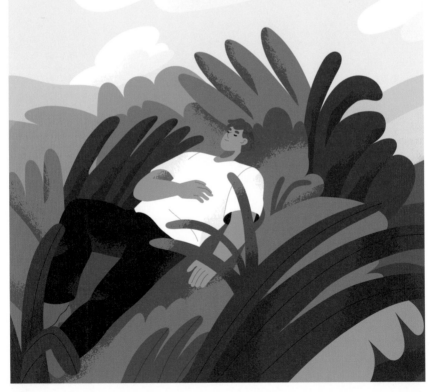

# EVERY DAY'S
# A SCHOOL DAY

Imposter syndrome and the general anxiety that makes you think "I can't do that" can make trying new things as an adult quite difficult. While children expect to be beginners at everything, as adults, we have a misplaced idea that we should already know how to do something, even if we're new to it.

Learning to drive at 40? Switching to a completely new career? Boiling an egg for the first time? It's okay to not know what you're doing. It's okay to ask for help and instruction. Own your beginner role and let the adult expectations drift away.

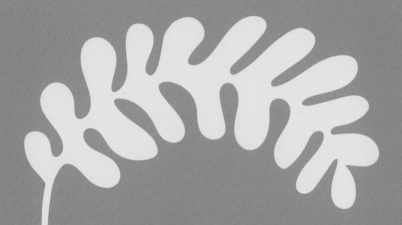

Allow yourself
to be a beginner

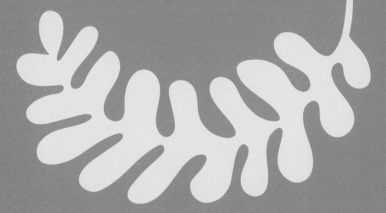

# LET KINDNESS RADIATE

We can't control other people's behaviour or responses, only our own. While at first this might seem inconvenient, it's actually very freeing. Choose to treat everyone, including yourself, with kindness and understanding. Even when others are being fractious, you can choose to respond calmly and kindly, deflecting rather than reflecting their negative energy.

When you treat everyone with kindness, you've done your best. How they choose to respond is wholly on them.

Be healthy and take care of yourself, but be happy with the beautiful things that make you, you.

Beyoncé

# CHAPTER THREE

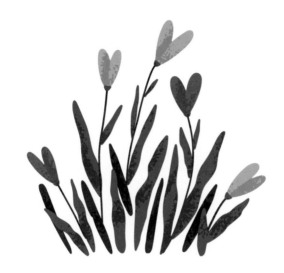

# TAKE GOOD CARE OF YOURSELF

Your mind and body are utterly intertwined. Taking care of your mind means taking care of your body, and vice versa, which is why the tips you'll find in this chapter are so important. Moving your body, sleeping well and eating healthily all positively influence your mood and mental resilience. This is great news, as a lot of the time it can feel easier to manage these things than an anxious brain. Read on to discover how you can care for your body to help ease anxiety.

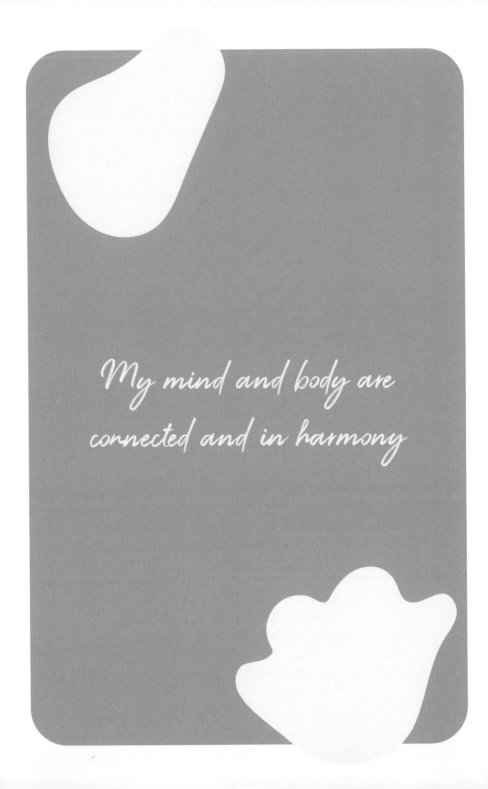

My mind and body are connected and in harmony

*If you've got it, flaunt it.
And if you don't got it?
Flaunt it. 'Cause what
are we even doing here if
we're not flaunting it?*

Mindy Kaling

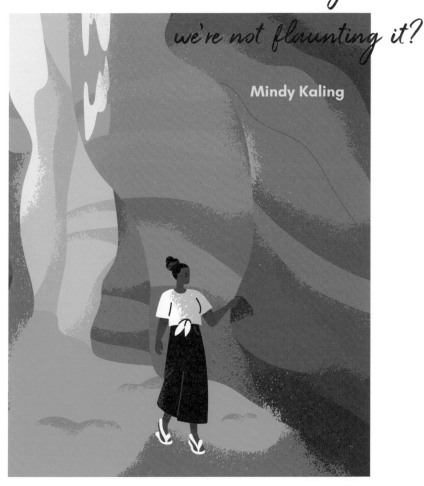

# GET A BETTER NIGHT'S SLEEP

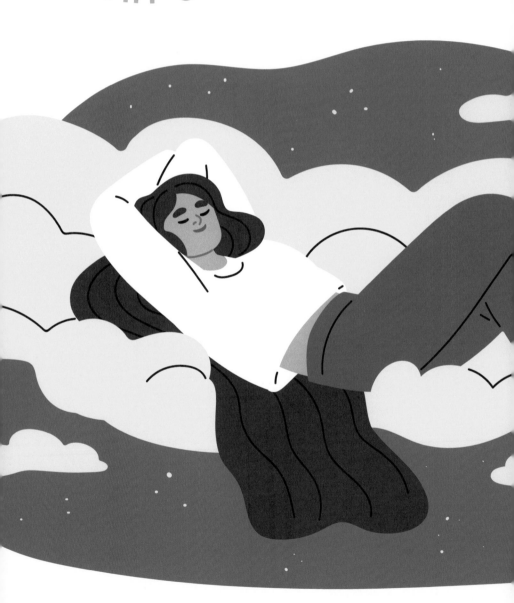

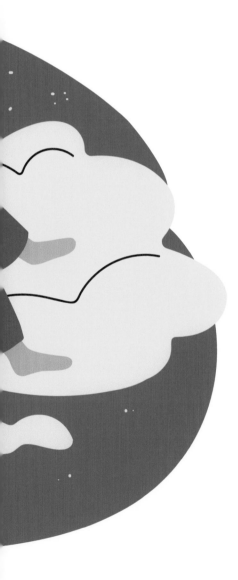

Starting your day following a good night's sleep is one of the cornerstones of good health, and, despite what many people think, you can't sleep more later to make up for poor sleep now. The irony here is that poor sleep can play into anxiety, and feeling anxious can contribute to poor sleep. But as good-quality sleep is vital for a healthy life, high cognitive function and a stable mood, it's a worthy cause.

Experts from around the world generally agree on these tips to improve your sleep quality:

- Get out into daylight, in the morning at least.

- Avoid caffeine after midday.

- Do something relaxing in the hour or two before bed, such as reading.

- Keep your phone and other electronic devices out of the bedroom, and preferably avoid them in the run-up to bedtime.

- Go to bed and wake up at roughly the same time every day.

- Do some light meditation (check the next tip, on page 86, for a great exercise).

# SHUTTING DOWN
# FOR THE DAY

To help you drift off to sleep,
try focusing on your mind-body
connection with this relaxing exercise:

1. Lie in bed and close your eyes.
2. Starting at your toes, imagine the
   muscles there gently switching off.
3. Draw your focus to your feet and
   lower legs, thinking of the muscles
   relaxing and powering down.
4. Continue slowly up the body,
   switching off your muscles as you go.
5. The sense of calm and relaxation
   this simple yet powerful exercise
   brings can send you to sleep
   before you've reached your head!

Almost everything will work again if you unplug it for a few minutes, including you.

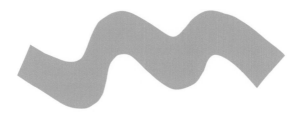

**Anne Lamott**

# HURRAH FOR HYDRATION!

Being dehydrated causes a lot of discomfort that you might not consider the result of dehydration at all. Not drinking enough water can contribute to low mood and low energy, neither of which helps ease anxiety. There's no need to carry a giant water bottle around with you all day, but do what you can to up your water intake if you think you're not getting enough. Great water sources include tea, soup and foods like watermelon and cucumber, as well as the stuff from the tap!

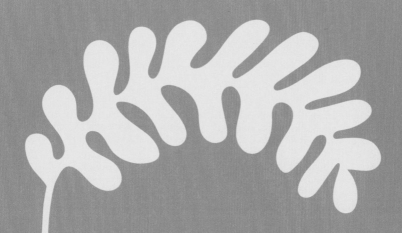

Pay attention to
the things that
matter to you

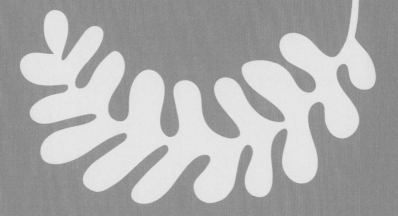

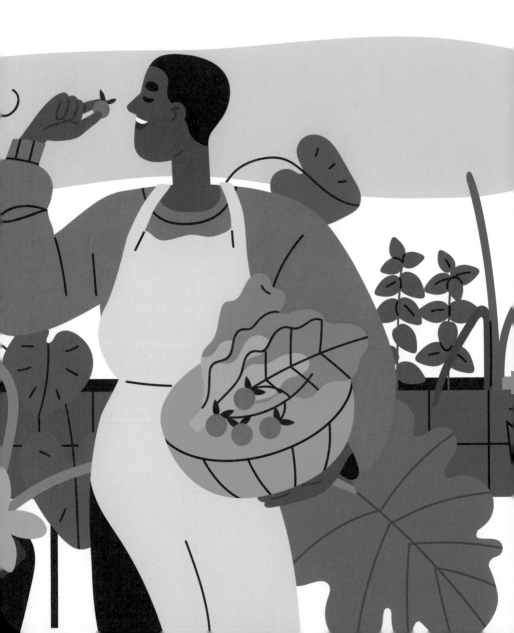

# YOU ARE
# WHAT YOU EAT

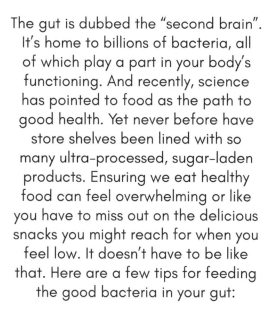

The gut is dubbed the "second brain". It's home to billions of bacteria, all of which play a part in your body's functioning. And recently, science has pointed to food as the path to good health. Yet never before have store shelves been lined with so many ultra-processed, sugar-laden products. Ensuring we eat healthy food can feel overwhelming or like you have to miss out on the delicious snacks you might reach for when you feel low. It doesn't have to be like that. Here are a few tips for feeding the good bacteria in your gut:

• Opt for whole foods: These are foods that are unprocessed or minimally processed, such as fruit and vegetables, beans and nuts, and whole grains, such as brown rice and oats.

• Cook from scratch: Find a recipe and make as much from scratch as possible. Short on time? Bulk cook and freeze things like pasta and curry sauces.

• Eat the rainbow: When planning a meal, start with the plant aspect of it and include multiple vegetables, each of a different colour. Different nutrients and vitamins create the colours, making this an effective way to eat a greater variety of good food.

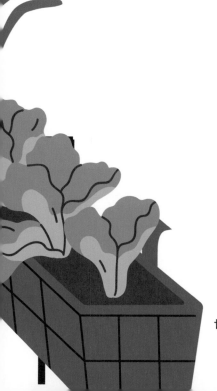

I am not a product of

my circumstances.

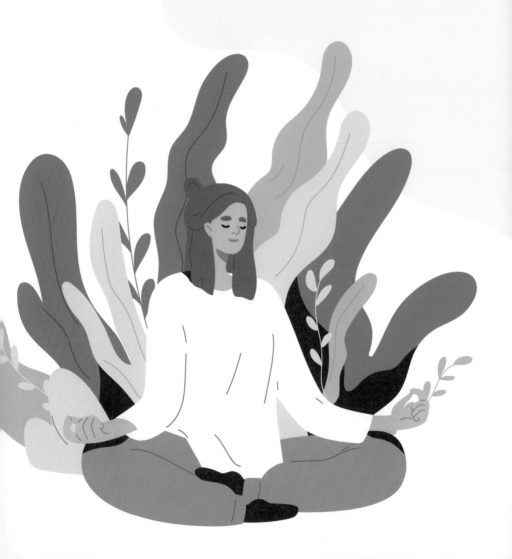

*I am a product of*

*my decisions.*

**Stephen R. Covey**

# YUMMY YOUTUBE

Stuck for what to cook? YouTube can be a great way to find delicious, healthy recipes and see how easy they are to make. Find out what main ingredients (such as vegetables) you have at home, then type "Quick [insert ingredient] dinner recipes" into the search bar.

Add other ingredients, such as "pasta" or "rice", into your search, and you'll be amazed at how many great dishes pop up for inspiration or the perfect meal for tonight. Doing research like this takes the pressure off and helps you make a healthy dinner while steering clear of junk food.

Nothing has transformed
my life more than
realizing that it's a
waste of time to evaluate
my worthiness by
weighing the reaction of
the people in the stands.

**Brené Brown**

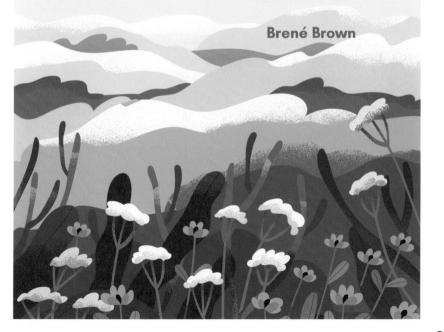

Absorb what is useful,
leave what is not

We always may
be what we might
have been.

Adelaide Anne Procter

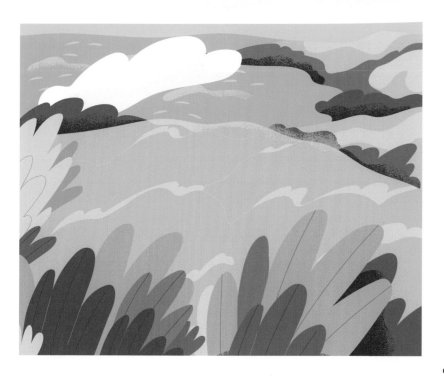

# CALM COOKING

Meal prep and cooking can be the most wonderful, mindful, anxiety-easing activities. Because you're doing something physical and mental simultaneously, there's little room for worries or anxieties to elbow in. Carve out some time to dedicate to making meals, whether it's batch cooking on a Sunday or calmly cooking every evening. As you work, notice the feeling of the knife chopping the veggies and the aromas of what you've got bubbling in the pan. Kitchens are spaces that allow you to tune in to all your senses at once.

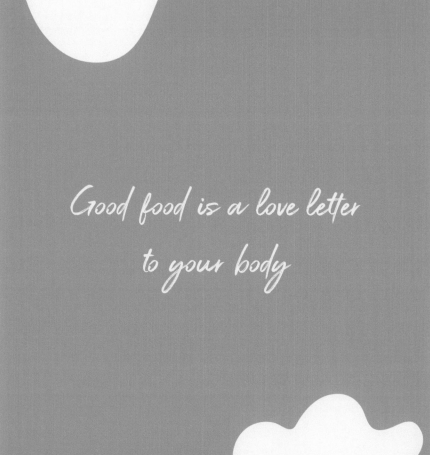

Good food is a love letter
to your body

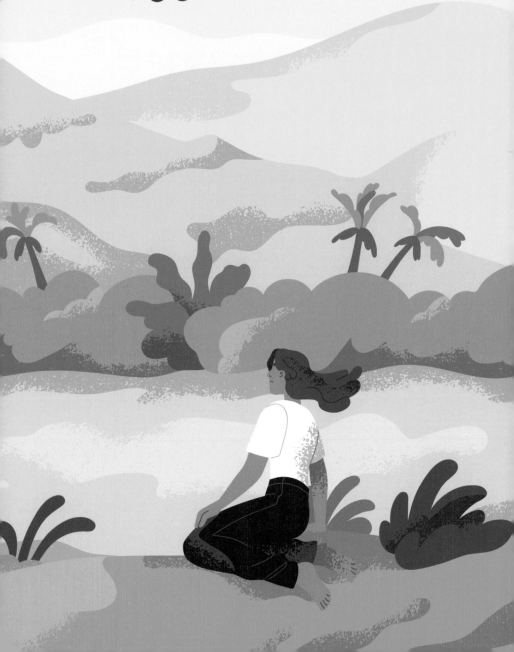

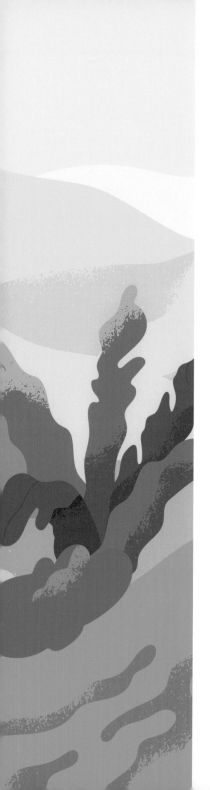

When anxiety steals the show, your body experiences it through tension, aches and even nausea. Strengthening the communication between your body and mind can bring you back into yourself, where anxiety will find it harder to take hold.

Gentle, considered activities are fantastic for infusing every part of your body with consciousness. They re-teach you how to "tune in" and feel what's going on. This isn't just useful for quelling anxiety; being able to "hear" your body means you'll be quicker to respond to its overall needs and warning signs. The following are examples of gentle movements that can help bring you back to your body and ease anxiety:

- Yoga: This ancient practice specifically works to connect your mind and body.

- Tai chi: A gentle, slow martial art, tai chi brings great awareness to how your body moves.

- Swimming: With your body fully supported in the water, swimming offers gentle exercise with rhythmic breathing and repetitive, almost meditative, motion.

# WORK
## ON YOUR
### STRENGTH

Strength training is essential for staying physically healthy into your later years, but it's great for easing anxiety too. Why? It doesn't take much training to feel tangibly stronger, where you can notice the added strength in daily activities, such as lifting heavier objects or climbing stairs. Seeing first-hand that your capabilities are boundless, and that you can become stronger, can provide a wonderful dose of self-confidence and increased feelings of resilience.

Bodyweight exercises, resistance bands, calisthenics or the good old gym are all great tools, so you can build strength in a way that suits you.

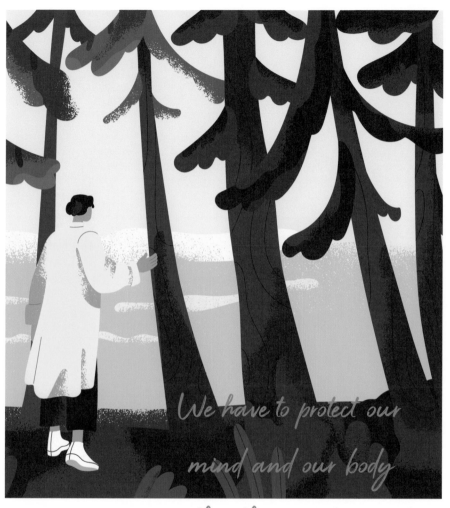

We have to protect our mind and our body rather than just go out there and do what the world wants us to do.

**Simone Biles**

# TAKE REGULAR
# MINI BREAKS

Prioritizing your mental and physical health during the working day is important. Focusing on work can see our bodies stuck in one position for hours, which can fatigue us and make us feel even worse. During the day, take regular mini breaks:

- Stand up, stretch and walk around if possible. Take the stairs to a bathroom on a different floor.
- Look far away, ideally out of a window at anything green and leafy.
- Take five deep inhales and exhales.
- Close your eyes for a moment.

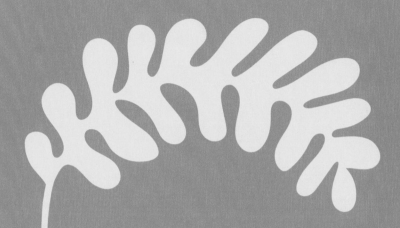

Let your body
move and your
heart will sing

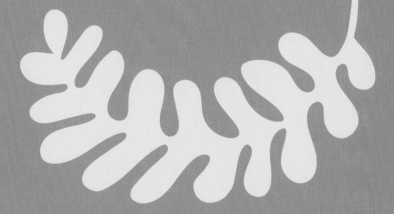

# AVOID ALCOHOL

Drinking alcohol can be a tricky activity when anxiety is hovering. The first drink may make you feel as though it's helping with anxiety, but that couldn't be further from the truth. Alcohol prevents us from dealing with our anxious thoughts in a healthy way and instead teaches us that we need it to get through dinners, events or other potentially anxiety-inducing occasions. It also hampers our sleep, and, as we saw on page 84, good sleep is a cornerstone of good mental health.

The "hangxiety" (hangover + anxiety) that can come after a night of drinking is a tough thing to handle, coupled with dehydration, nausea and a headache. Cutting down on or giving up alcohol entirely can do wonders for easing anxiety. Practising a lighter intake can increase your self-confidence and reveal that you don't need it to get through anything – you're resilient enough just as you are.

I've seen people go from
the darkest moments in
their lives to living a
happy, fulfilling life.

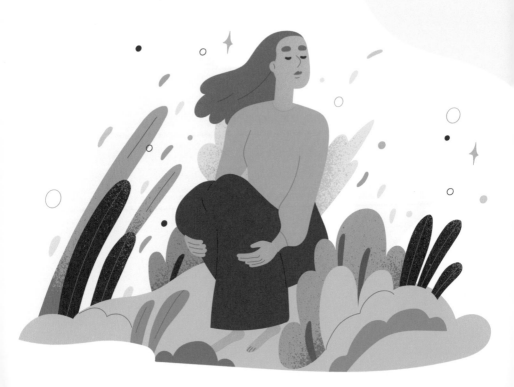

*You can do it too.*

*I believe in you.*

**Sophie Turner**

# RECONNECTING WITH NATURE

Both green spaces, filled with trees and fields, and blue spaces, comprising lakes, rivers and seascapes, bring with them an inherent sense of calm and peace to the mind and body. Natural environments are fantastic for balancing your mental health, and you don't have to live rurally to experience this relief. Take some time every day to go for a short walk, run or bike ride in a natural environment. Head to a park or lake and really focus on the natural elements you see, such as trees, birds and flowers.

There is no hurry.

We shall get there some day.

**A. A. Milne**

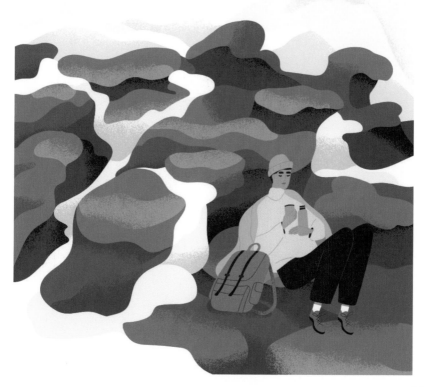

# FOREST BATHING

Known as shinrin-yoku in Japanese, forest bathing is the ancient practice of mindfully spending time among trees. In our modern lives, it's even more crucial to take time out, perhaps on a weekend or day off, and leave behind the incessant chatter of the online world, spending time in nature instead. To practise forest bathing:

- Seek out a woodland.
- Leave behind headphones and silence your phone.
- Amble among the trees.
- Sit quietly, taking in the sights and sounds of the wood.
- Reflect on how you feel afterwards. Soothed?

It's okay to slow down and take the time you need

# SHAKE IT OUT

While gentler forms of exercise and movement can be calming and restorative, giving yourself permission to let it all spill out can be invigorating and life-affirming. That's why dance and dance-based workouts are so joyful and uplifting. You can pursue some dance for grace and technique, creating fine-tuned connections between your mind and body. Other forms are more carefree, fun-packed and heart-rate rising. Here are some of the specific benefits of dance.

## Music
With pumping music, many types of dance allow you to free your mind and body through movement and sound, moving instinctually to the beat.

## Movement
Dance is fundamentally a form of self-expression, giving you permission to move as freely as you like.

## Sociability
Feeling inhibited is common before taking up dance, but the beauty of this activity is the ebbing of self-consciousness, as everyone around you is also dancing. This frees you from anxiety and might offer up a whole bunch of new friends!

Great dancers are not great because of their technique, they are great because of their passion.

Martha Graham

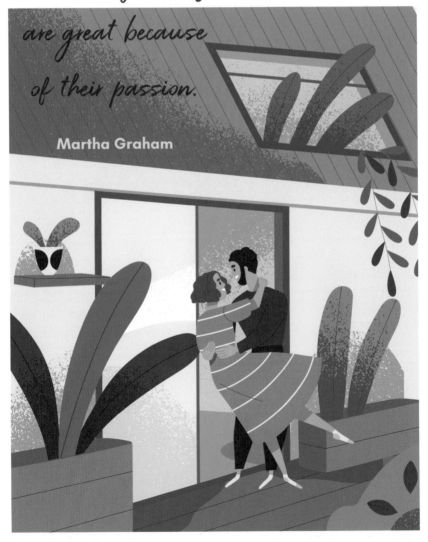

# STRETCH
# IT OUT

Whether you sit at a desk or work on your feet, the body benefits from doing as cats do: stretching often. Tension builds throughout the day in different muscles, especially if you're still for hours. It's only when you begin to stretch that you realize quite how much you needed it... and just how good it feels. Tension release not only helps the body, but is also a mindful practice that soothes the brain. The internet is a great place to find stretching videos that you can do at home, and some yoga studios offer dedicated stretching classes too.

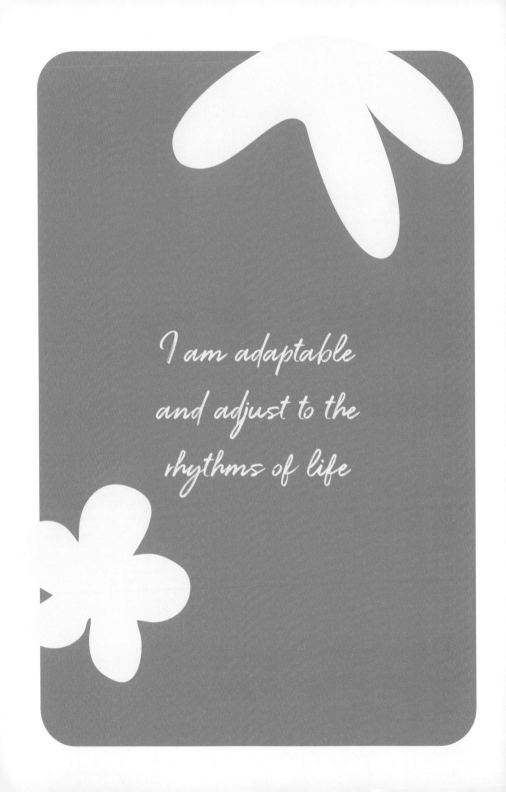

I am adaptable
and adjust to the
rhythms of life

# BUILD SUSTAINABLE HABITS

Taking care of your body and mind is a holistic, continual, lifelong process. Trying to attain a "perfect" self-care routine is neither sustainable nor very kind to yourself. So, eschew "gurus" or "morning routines" that you might see online, and instead build in self-care, little by little, in a way that suits you and your needs. Starting small and manageable is the key to building better habits, rather than deciding that, from tomorrow, you'll always drink plenty of water, sleep like a baby and eat purely organic.

Follow your instincts.
That is where true wisdom
manifests itself.

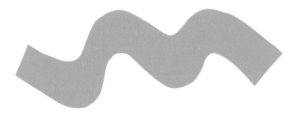

**Oprah Winfrey**

# CHAPTER FOUR

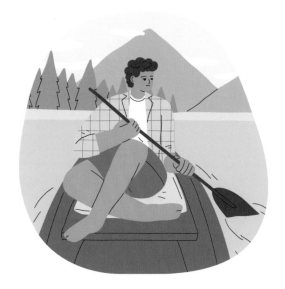

# A CALMER FUTURE

Managing anxiety in the long term means setting yourself up for success by knowing how to handle the threat when it strikes. While anxious moments are a normal part of life, they can sometimes knock you off your feet when they arrive. Having techniques you can call on in the moment will help you ride the wave calmly and proactively. Simply recognizing anxiety is the first step, while knowing that you have the power to manage it is the second. Read on to learn how you can begin taking it in stride...

# VISUALIZE A BETTER EXPERIENCE

Visualizing how your life will look with less anxiety can help you see that this outcome is truly possible. Follow these simple steps:

- Find a comfortable, quiet place to sit.
- Consider an upcoming situation that is likely to bring about anxious feelings.
- Close your eyes and take a few slow, deep breaths, before letting your breathing settle.
- In your mind, walk through the situation; picture yourself at ease, smiling and seeing that everything is going well.
- Picture the small things: colourful scenes, pleasant scents and the slow, easy breath in your body.
- Remain in this visualization for a while, before opening your eyes and noticing how you feel.

It's okay if the visualization didn't reduce your anxious thoughts straight away – it's a journey, so visualizing regularly is key.

# TAKE BACK CONTROL

Anxiety can arise from feeling like you're not able to do something competently. An antidote to this is to brush up your skills. You can't learn everything, but reminding yourself what you can learn will get you a long way.

- Going to a country where the people speak a different language? Take a basic language class.
- Lost when it comes to DIY? Learn from YouTube.
- Worried you can't keep up with your kids? Start running, or join a workout class.

There's always a way to increase your knowledge and skills.

Nothing we learn in
this world is ever wasted
and I have come to
the conclusion that
practically nothing we
do ever stands by itself.

**Eleanor Roosevelt**

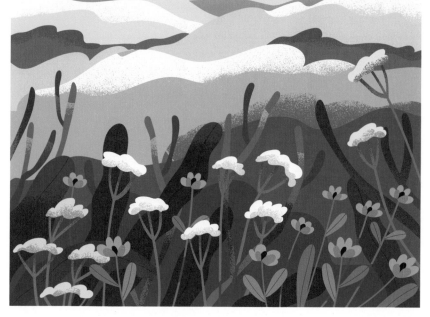

# PHONE
# A FRIEND

When we start feeling anxious, we tend to only look inwards. We worry about what people will think or say about us. To insert a thought-breaker, think of a friend whom you haven't spoken to in a while, or who might be going through a challenge of their own, be it a new job or a difficult situation. Call them up and make it your number-one priority to improve their day. Listen to whatever's going on with them, ask questions about their life and do your best to make them laugh. You'll leave the conversation feeling uplifted at having helped someone else.

I belong wherever
I decide I belong

# RELEASE NEGATIVE THOUGHTS

Anxious thoughts are often only powerful when they stay trapped inside our heads, like big fish circling a little pond. One of the most popular treatments for anxiety is talking therapy, which ranges from counselling to CBT (cognitive behavioural therapy). Talking to someone, particularly an impartial person who isn't normally part of your life, can have a hugely beneficial effect. Where to find talking therapies:

- See your doctor for confidential advice.
- In some places, you can self-refer to CBT or talking therapy.
- Look for self-help tools and CBT courses online.
- Seek out private counsellors and therapists.

It might take effort to find a method or person who is the right fit for you, but persevering is worthwhile. Talking therapies can last as long as you need, and you can revisit these methods throughout your life.

*If everything*

*was perfect*

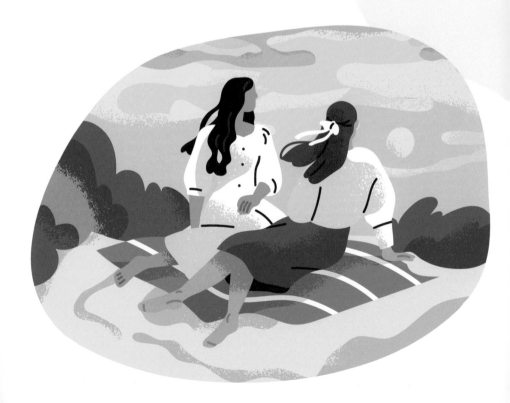

then you would
never learn and you
would never grow

# DISTANCE YOURSELF FROM YOUR PHONE

You might only realize you're missing your phone when you reach out for it and it's not there. For many of us, picking up our phones happens on autopilot. And yet, social media, the news and even our inboxes can be a strong source of anxiety. To build greater self-awareness and moderate phone usage, try one or two of these tactics:

- Turn your screen to greyscale.
- Leave it in another room.
- Put it on silent.
- Download a focus app that incentivizes not using your phone.

Our freedom can
be measured by the
number of things we
can walk away from.

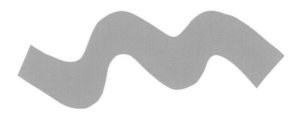

**Vernon Howard**

# THE POWER OF
# THE BREATH

Using breathing for anxiety reduction is a practice that is thousands of years old, and modern science backs it up. When we breathe calmly and deeply, our nervous system relaxes, helping us know we are safe. Try this classic breathing exercise, called 4–7–8 breathing:

1. Sit comfortably and inhale deeply for four seconds.
2. Hold the breath for seven seconds.
3. Exhale slowly for eight seconds.
4. Repeat five times.

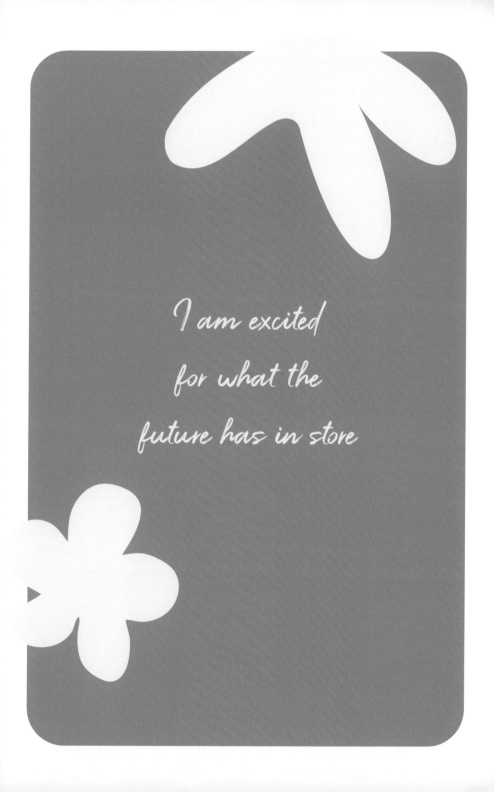

I am excited
for what the
future has in store

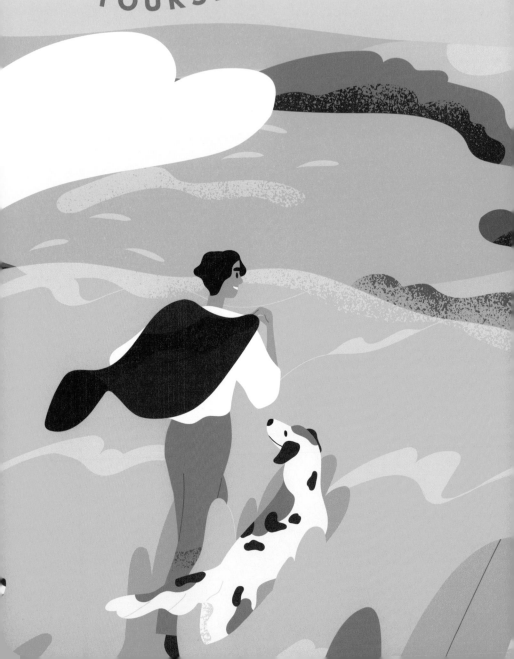

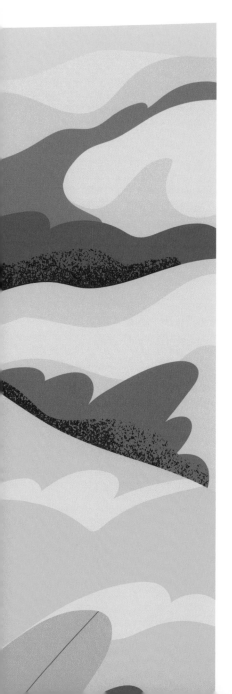

You can take all the warm baths and beautiful walks you like, but if you put everyone else before yourself, anxiety may stay close by. We learn to respect ourselves by honouring our values and standing by what we believe in and who we are. It's not an overnight process, but here are a couple of things you can bring into your life that will help to generate self-respect.

### Be you, not them

A great exercise in self-respect is to accept who you are and who you are not. We may often find ourselves trying to be like someone else, or trying to like something that others like. Great empowerment comes from pausing and saying, "Actually, that's not for me."

### Finish your sentence

If you find yourself being interrupted, do you immediately stop talking and give the floor to the other person? Try responding with "Please let me finish." It can feel intimidating at first, but with a confident smile, chances are you can finish what you were saying. Respecting your own voice helps to build self-respect and wider authority.

# REDUCE THE OVERWHELM

There's a lot of noise in modern life – sometimes literally. If anxiety is rising and you're in a place where there are competing sounds, try going somewhere quieter. Although we might not think of it this way, listening to something while performing a task is a form of multitasking, even if it's music, the radio or other conversations. Simplifying the load on your senses by going somewhere quiet or turning the music off can reduce cognitive overwhelm.

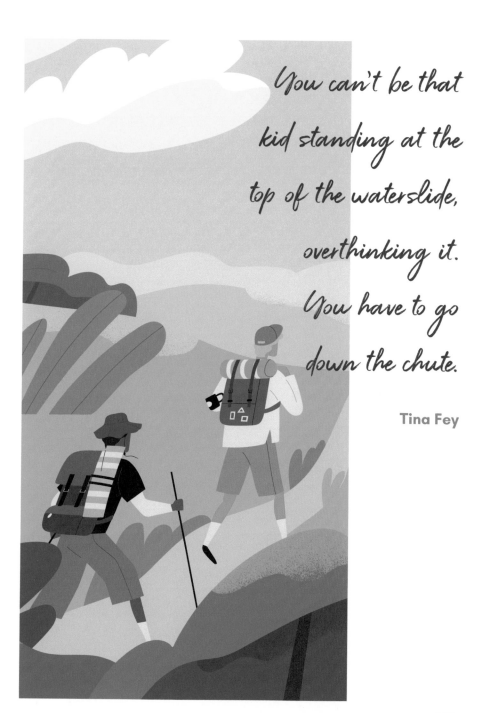

You can't be that kid standing at the top of the waterslide, overthinking it. You have to go down the chute.

**Tina Fey**

# EMBRACE SOOTHING SOUNDS

Just like turning down the noise can reduce feelings of overwhelm, embracing calming sounds can increase a sense of relaxation. Using a sound to relax is an ancient technique, but one that's still frequently practised today. You could look for sound bath sessions nearby, listen to one online or simply choose a favourite relaxing album to listen to. Try to keep this sound session at the same time every week (or day, if you have time). Consistency helps build sustainable habits.

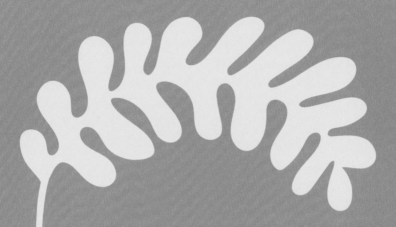

Embrace your
feelings fully

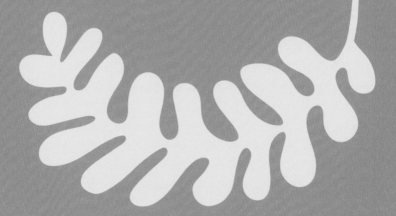

# MAKE TIME
# FOR MEDITATION

There are examples of meditation throughout this book (for example, on page 86), but it cannot be stressed enough how powerful a tool this is for managing anxiety. Meditation is not about clearing your mind of thoughts. Instead, it's a long-term practice that allows you to let go of thoughts easily when they arise, helping to lessen negativity. Meditation can be challenging to get into, especially when we're used to being so busy. Consistency, rather than duration, is key. Ten minutes a day, regularly, can have numerous benefits.

### Building a meditation practice

- **Learn:** Read about the benefits of meditation to get a clear picture of why this practice will help you.
- **Support:** Find an app or class that can teach you the basics and provide guided meditations.
- **Time:** Stick to a consistent time every day for your meditation practice.
- **Kindness:** Missing a day doesn't mean you should give up. Be kind to yourself and simply pick it up again the next day.
- **Journal:** Writing things down gives them greater sticking power. Briefly journal about your meditation after each session.

Take chances, make
mistakes. That's
how you grow.

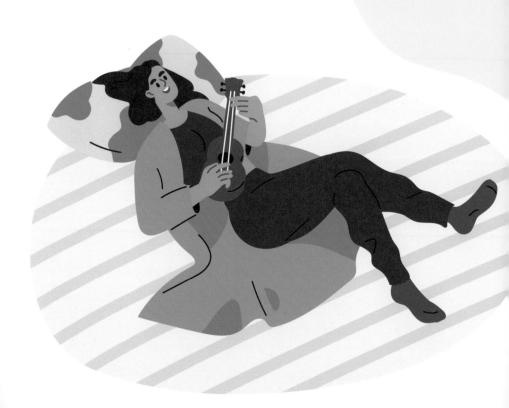

Pain nourishes your courage. You have to fail in order to practice being brave.

**Mary Tyler Moore**

# CELEBRATE YOURSELF

Experiencing anxiety can make you feel like you always have to strive to do better, but actually, you've already accomplished so many great things. Reminding yourself of – and celebrating – your strengths and achievements is a powerful technique of self-support that helps build resilience and self-respect.

Weekly, monthly or biannually, write a list of your strengths and achievements. Small things, such as helping a friend move house, are just as valuable as finishing a degree, learning a new skill or getting your dream job.

*Meanings are not determined by situations, but we determine ourselves by the meanings we give situations.*

**Alfred Adler**

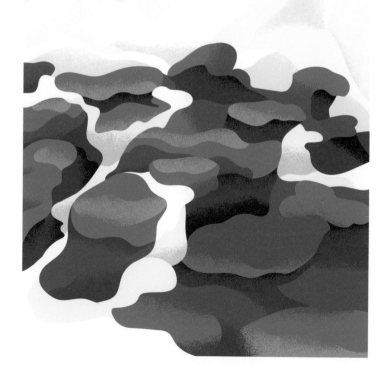

# YOU ARE WHO YOU SURROUND YOURSELF WITH

The people around you can have a much greater effect on what you do and feel than you might think. Working and socializing with people who support, uplift and challenge you can have a beneficial influence. Consider who you spend lots of time with: do they respect your boundaries, provide support and leave you feeling positive? These people are gold. If you regularly interact with people who leave you feeling unsure, like you're walking on eggshells, or who actively upset you, it's time to create some distance.

I fill my life with
supportive people and
I support them in return

# BUILDING A
# SUPPORT NETWORK

Everyone needs people they can turn to for support. Your network doesn't have to be huge; instead, it can be made up of people who offer different functions and at differing levels of closeness. Having people you can reach out to regularly means you can express yourself truthfully and ask for help. Without a good support system, loneliness and anxiety can seep in. Here are a few examples of where you can find your support network:

- **Friends:** Old or new, these are the people you can tell private things and call at a moment's notice. Consider who you'd go to for a hug or who you'd send a hilarious meme to.
- **Colleagues:** Once removed from your personal life, colleagues can offer more objective advice. They can also be great for development support.
- **Acquaintances:** Joining clubs, classes or charitable endeavours can boost social connections and provide a different kind of support – one that comes from doing a certain activity with people who share an interest or value.

Remember, support works both ways. By growing your network, you're helping others grow theirs.

Surround yourself
with people and things
that inspire you. Learn
everything you can.

**Jameela Jamil**

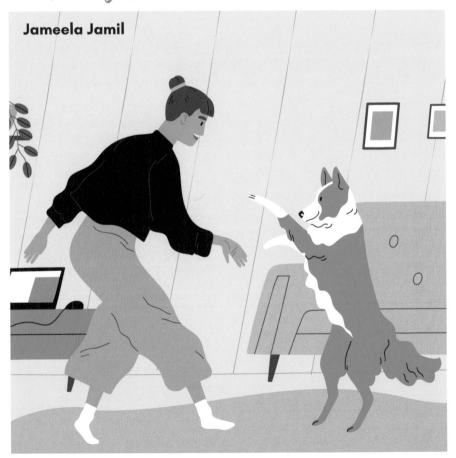

# GIVE YOURSELF PERMISSION TO PRIORITIZE

You're already prioritizing every day. The question is, are you prioritizing the things that are right for you?

Giving yourself permission to prioritize things in a way that respects your values is a powerful tool to ease anxiety and reduce internal conflict. It's not as simple as making a numbered list, but if you write down what you do in a week, and then see which things fall into which category below, you may find your priorities aren't focused where you'd like them to be...

- Social/Family
- Work
- Personal Development/Hobbies
- Relaxation/Entertainment

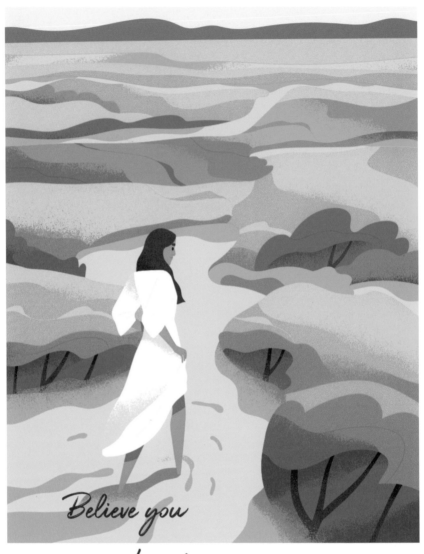

Believe you
can and you're
halfway there.

**Theodore Roosevelt**

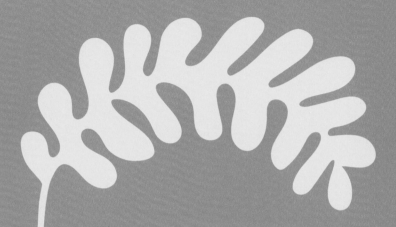

Great
opportunities
are flowing
towards me

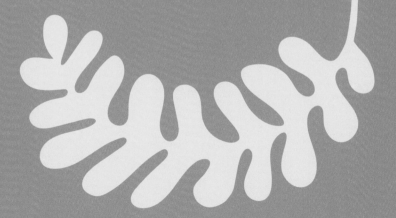

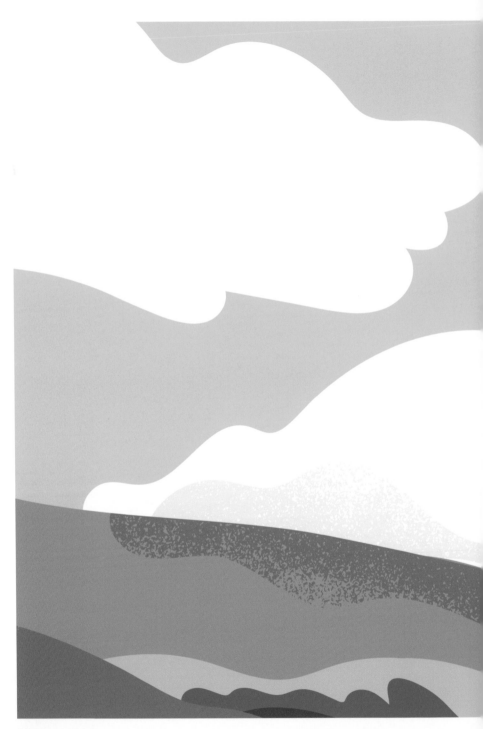

# CONCLUSION

This wild adventure called life is filled with unknowables. But even though this thought can sometimes seem overwhelming, remember: taking comfort in the tips and techniques throughout this book will help to ease the anxiety that may have been stopping you from reaching your full potential, so you can embrace everything your future holds.

By easing your anxiety (if and when it comes calling), you can reignite the power you have within, and you no longer need to listen to that tired, old, negative voice. Through kindness, self-love and respect, and by showing up for yourself every day, you can journey onwards, appreciating the many joys in life, both big and small.

So, breathe deeply and remember to reconnect to yourself often. You are filled with potential and you have everything you need within to live a wonderful life. Good luck... and enjoy!

# How to Be Present: Embrace the Art of Mindfulness to Discover Peace and Joy Every Day

Sophie Golding

Paperback

978-1-80007-395-1

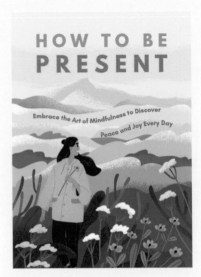

**Discover the art of being present. Filled with simple advice and inspiring quotes, this book will show you how to appreciate each moment, helping you to live more every day.**

To experience happiness and fulfilment day to day, you don't need to change your life – you simply need to be present in it.

Through a collection of easy-to-follow tips, this book will show you how to shift your mindset and live more fully in the moment. Over the course of its chapters, you will learn how to:

- Incorporate mindfulness practices into your day
- Reduce feelings of stress and anxiety
- Strengthen the connection between your mind and body
- Find joy, wonder and gratitude in every day

There are so many moments worth cherishing in our daily lives, and when you focus on the now, they're yours to find. So dive into these beautiful pages and give yourself the gift of being present every day.

# How to Live Your Best Life: Live a Life You Love and Find Joy and Fulfilment Every Day

Sophie Golding

Paperback

978-1-80007-936-6

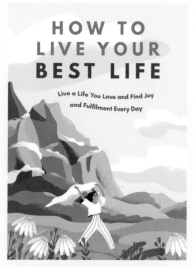

**Live your life to the fullest! Filled with thoughtful advice and inspiring quotes and affirmations, this book will show you how to envision your best, happiest life and make it reality.**

Your best life is yours to define. Whether it means reaching for your dreams, finding a sense of purpose or making more time for the things you love, it's whatever makes you feel like the very best version of yourself.

Learn how to:

- Visualize what your best life looks like for you
- Identify your core values and align your life with them
- Adjust your mindset with small changes and habits to stay motivated and happy
- Find peace within yourself and nurture self-love

We are at our happiest when what we do matches up with who we are, so dive into these beautiful pages to begin your journey towards a life of joy and fulfilment.

Have you enjoyed this book?
If so, why not write a review on your favourite website?

If you're interested in finding out
more about our books, find us on Facebook
at **Summersdale Publishers**, on Twitter/X
at **@Summersdale** and on Instagram and
TikTok at **@summersdalebooks** and get
in touch. We'd love to hear from you!

Thanks very much for buying
this Summersdale book.

**www.summersdale.com**

## Image credits